Talking
JOURNAL

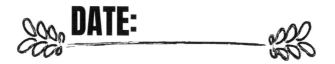 **DATE:** _____

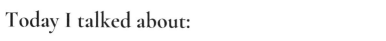

Today I talked about:

Something I found challenging:

Something I found helpful:

Something I want to remember:

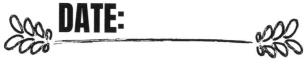 **DATE:** _____

Today I talked about:

Something I found challenging:

Something I found helpful:

Something I want to remember:

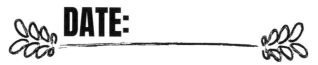 **DATE:** _____

Today I talked about:

Something I found challenging:

Something I found helpful:

Something I want to remember:

 **DATE:** _____

Today I talked about:

Something I found challenging:

Something I found helpful:

Something I want to remember:

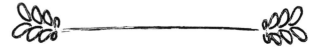

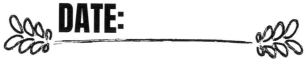 **DATE:** _____

Today I talked about:

Something I found challenging:

Something I found helpful:

Something I want to remember:

 ———————

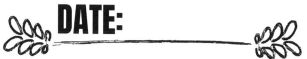 **DATE:** _____

Today I talked about:

Something I found challenging:

Something I found helpful:

Something I want to remember:

 ———————

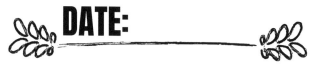 **DATE:** _____

Today I talked about:

Something I found challenging:

Something I found helpful:

Something I want to remember:

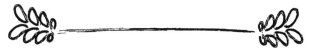

DATE: _____

Today I talked about:

Something I found challenging:

Something I found helpful:

Something I want to remember:

 **DATE:** _____

Today I talked about:

Something I found challenging:

Something I found helpful:

Something I want to remember:

 **DATE:** _____

Today I talked about:

Something I found challenging:

Something I found helpful:

Something I want to remember:

 ———————

 **DATE:** _____

Today I talked about:

Something I found challenging:

Something I found helpful:

Something I want to remember:

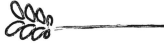

DATE: _____

Today I talked about:

Something I found challenging:

Something I found helpful:

Something I want to remember:

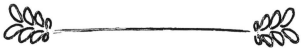

DATE: _____

Today I talked about:

Something I found challenging:

Something I found helpful:

Something I want to remember:

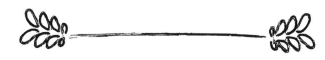

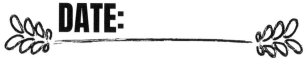

DATE: _____

Today I talked about:

Something I found challenging:

Something I found helpful:

Something I want to remember:

 **DATE:** _____

Today I talked about:

Something I found challenging:

Something I found helpful:

Something I want to remember:

 _____

DATE: _____

Today I talked about:

Something I found challenging:

Something I found helpful:

Something I want to remember:

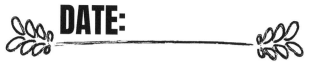 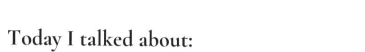

DATE: _____

Today I talked about:

Something I found challenging:

Something I found helpful:

Something I want to remember:

DATE: _____

Today I talked about:

Something I found challenging:

Something I found helpful:

Something I want to remember:

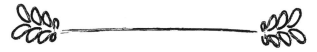

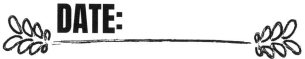

DATE: _____

Today I talked about:

Something I found challenging:

Something I found helpful:

Something I want to remember:

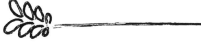

 **DATE:** _____

Today I talked about:

Something I found challenging:

Something I found helpful:

Something I want to remember:

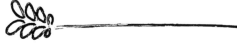

 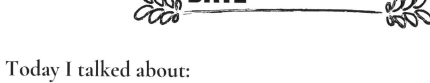 **DATE:** _____

Today I talked about:

Something I found challenging:

Something I found helpful:

Something I want to remember:

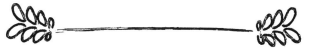

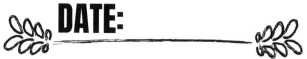 **DATE:** _____

Today I talked about:

Something I found challenging:

Something I found helpful:

Something I want to remember:

 _____

 **DATE:** _____

Today I talked about:

Something I found challenging:

Something I found helpful:

Something I want to remember:

 **DATE:** _____

Today I talked about:

Something I found challenging:

Something I found helpful:

Something I want to remember:

 **DATE:** _____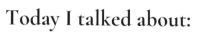

Today I talked about:

Something I found challenging:

Something I found helpful:

Something I want to remember:

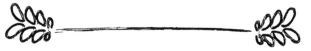

 **DATE:** _____

Today I talked about:

Something I found challenging:

Something I found helpful:

Something I want to remember:

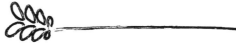

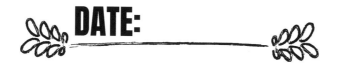

DATE: _____

Today I talked about:

Something I found challenging:

Something I found helpful:

Something I want to remember:

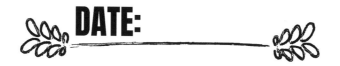 **DATE:** _____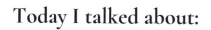

Today I talked about:

Something I found challenging:

Something I found helpful:

Something I want to remember:

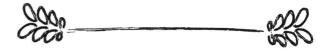

 **DATE:** _____

Today I talked about:

Something I found challenging:

Something I found helpful:

Something I want to remember:

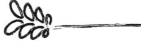

 **DATE:** _____

Today I talked about:

Something I found challenging:

Something I found helpful:

Something I want to remember:

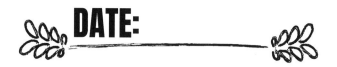
DATE: _____

Today I talked about:

Something I found challenging:

Something I found helpful:

Something I want to remember:

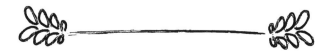

 **DATE:** _____

Today I talked about:

Something I found challenging:

Something I found helpful:

Something I want to remember:

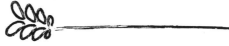

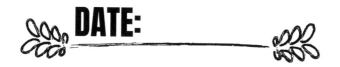 **DATE:** _____

Today I talked about:

Something I found challenging:

Something I found helpful:

Something I want to remember:

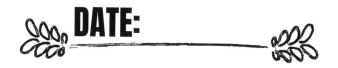

DATE: _____

Today I talked about:

Something I found challenging:

Something I found helpful:

Something I want to remember:

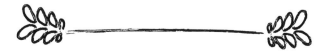

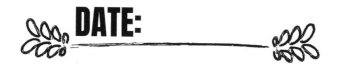

DATE: _____

Today I talked about:

Something I found challenging:

Something I found helpful:

Something I want to remember:

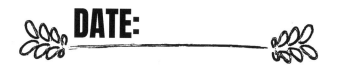

DATE: _____

Today I talked about:

Something I found challenging:

Something I found helpful:

Something I want to remember:

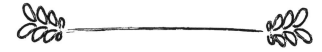

DATE: _____

Today I talked about:

Something I found challenging:

Something I found helpful:

Something I want to remember:

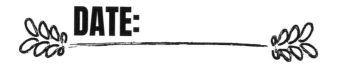

DATE: _____

Today I talked about:

Something I found challenging:

Something I found helpful:

Something I want to remember:

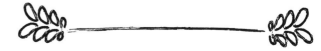

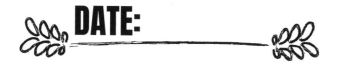 **DATE:** _____

Today I talked about:

Something I found challenging:

Something I found helpful:

Something I want to remember:

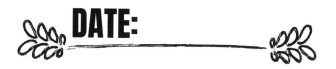

DATE: _____

Today I talked about:

Something I found challenging:

Something I found helpful:

Something I want to remember:

 **DATE:** _____

Today I talked about:

Something I found challenging:

Something I found helpful:

Something I want to remember:

 ———————

DATE: _____

Today I talked about:

Something I found challenging:

Something I found helpful:

Something I want to remember:

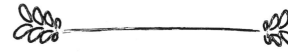

DATE: _____

Today I talked about:

Something I found challenging:

Something I found helpful:

Something I want to remember:

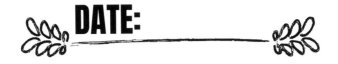

DATE: _____

Today I talked about:

Something I found challenging:

Something I found helpful:

Something I want to remember:

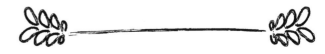

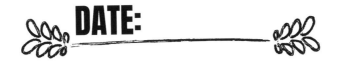

DATE: _____

Today I talked about:

Something I found challenging:

Something I found helpful:

Something I want to remember:

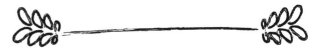

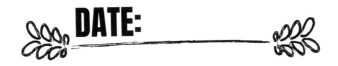

DATE: _____

Today I talked about:

Something I found challenging:

Something I found helpful:

Something I want to remember:

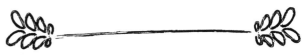

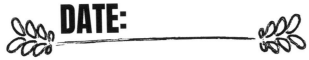
DATE: _____

Today I talked about:

Something I found challenging:

Something I found helpful:

Something I want to remember:

DATE: _____

Today I talked about:

Something I found challenging:

Something I found helpful:

Something I want to remember:

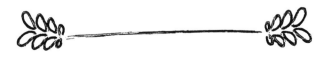

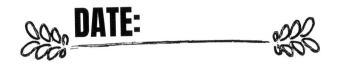
DATE: _____

Today I talked about:

Something I found challenging:

Something I found helpful:

Something I want to remember:

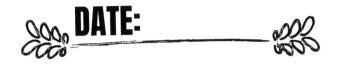

DATE: _____

Today I talked about:

Something I found challenging:

Something I found helpful:

Something I want to remember:

Made in the USA
Columbia, SC
14 December 2024

49444317R00057